Baking Soda
Earth Friendly
Natural Cleaning

---

65 Recipes

By: Samantha Miller

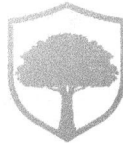

CLADD
PUBLISHING

Cladd Publishing Inc.
USA

This publication is designed to provide accurate information regarding the
subject matter covered. It is sold with the understanding that neither the
author nor the publisher is providing medical, legal or other professional
advice or services. Always seek advice from a competent professional
before using any of the information in this book. The author and the
publisher specifically disclaim any liability that is incurred from the use or
application of the contents of this book.

Baking Soda Earth Friendly Natural Cleaning: 65 Recipes

ISBN 978-1-946881-40-3 (e-book)
ISBN 978-1-946881-39-7 (paperback)

Contents

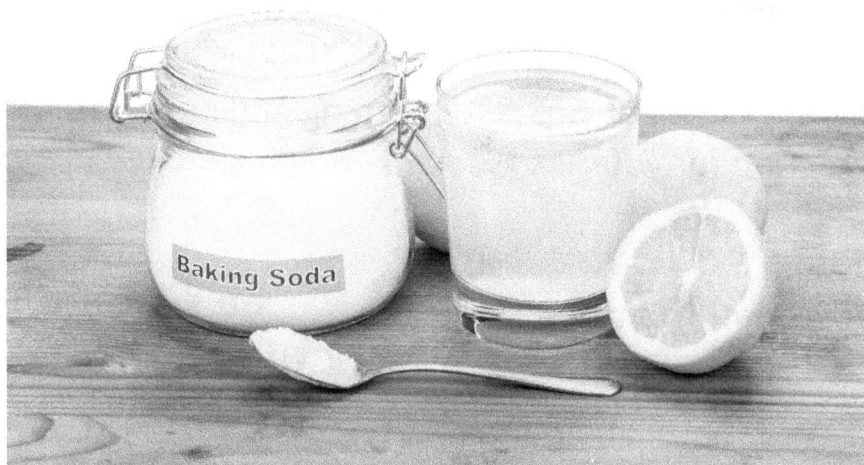

Cleaning Power of Baking Soda

Baking Soda, also known as Sodium Bicarbonate, is a natural occurring mineral. It is absolutely one of the safest, and most versatile substances in the world. You will learn how to use baking soda to provide a Super-Charged cleaning and deodorizing solution for your everyday needs.

Learn How to Clean:
- Bathrooms
- Kitchens
- Fabrics, and bedding
- Remove water marks
- Septic tanks
- Unclog drains and pips
- Deodorize entire home, vehicle and outdoor equipment
- Remove stains from floors, concrete, upholstery and carpet
- Extinguish grease fires
- Gently clean marble, wood, walls and Formica
- Restore shine
- Make homemade spackle
- Clean jewelry, brass, chrome and stainless steal

- Remove grime from anything
- Super-charge laundry cleaning
- Safely clean delicate items, mouth gear and brushes
- Carwash solutions
- Corrosion free De-icer for driveways and sidewalks
- And much more....

How It Was Used in Ancient Times

The use of sodium bicarbonate, extends thousands of years into Ancient Egypt; where it was a staple in everyday life. They used it to form paint for their hieroglyphics, to clean teeth, as a powerful cleaning agent, to treat all types of wounds, and to dry out bodies for the mummification process.

The Magical Cleaning Power

Baking Soda is natural, frugal, and downright amazing. It's gentle, safe and effective as a cleaner for glass, brass, chrome, steel, enamel and plastics. Baking soda is non-toxic, unlike many other household cleaners.

It is safe to use around children and pets. If you want to save the planet, this is a great way to start.

Baking soda is perfect for cleaning food preparation surfaces, microwaves, ovens, pots and pans, and your good silver. its tremendous cleaning power goes beyond the kitchen in to the bathrooms. It easily handles sinks, tubs, tile, drains and even teeth without scratching. It is already being used in factories to clean large machinery and commercial kitchen equipment.

Baking Soda Cleaning Characteristics:

- non-toxic
- Eco-Friendly
- Frugal
- Mildly basic (alkaline) buffer
- Gentle abrasive (non-scratching)
- Effervescent
- Neutralizer
- Reacts with dirt and grease to form a cleanser
- And many more

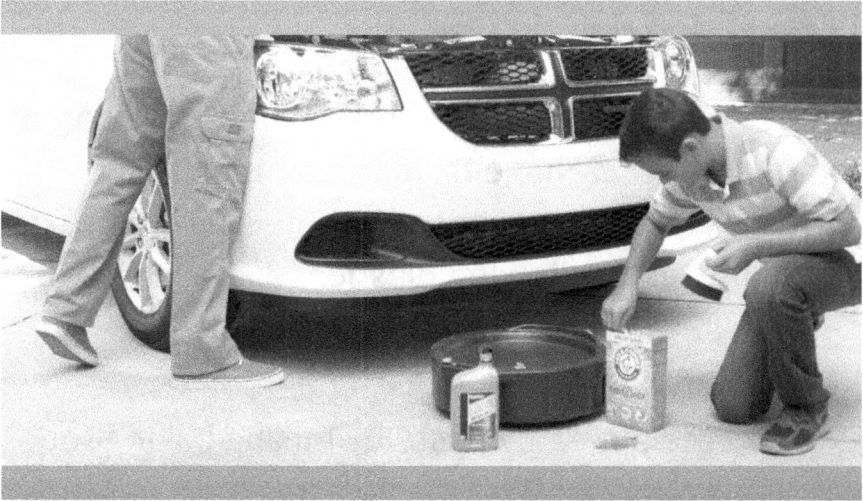

Auto Care

Dead Bugs

It may be one of the most best cleaning solution to remove insect carnage from unpainted car surfaces like bumpers and windshields. Also use on headlights and yellowing plastic.

HOW TO:

- Create a creamy paste by mixing baking soda and water together.
- Make as much or as little of this paste as you would like.
- Add a little dish soap.
- Gently scrub the areas of concern with a sponge, microfiber or washcloth.
- Rinse well.

Car Wash

A perfect solution for cleaning entire car, tires, windows, floor mats and vinyl seats.

HOW TO:

- Add ½ cup of baking soda in a half gallon of warm water.
- Add a squirt of dish soap.

- Gently scrub the entire car.
- Rinse well.
- Dry with cloth or microfiber towel.

Deodorizing Cars

HOW TO:
- Sprinkle baking soda directly on the fabric seats and carpets.
- Let sit for 1-24 hours.
- Vacuum up the baking soda.

Neutralize battery acid corrosion

The ability of baking soda to neutralize acid can save even the most corroded battery terminals.

HOW TO:
- Mix six tablespoons of baking soda into four cups of water.
- pour the mixture over the corrosion.
- Let it to sit for five minutes.
- Scrub with a toothbrush.
- then rinse or wipe it off.

Tires & Hubcaps

How To:
- Mix one-half cup baking soda.
- 1 tablespoon of dish soap.
- 2 cups of warm water into a small bowl.
- Use a soft sponge or towel to gently scrub the tires and hubcaps.
- Rinse well.

Magical De-Icer

This recipe works wonders on your icing sidewalk, deck, porch and driveway.

How To:
- Scatter baking soda on icy sidewalks.
- Done.

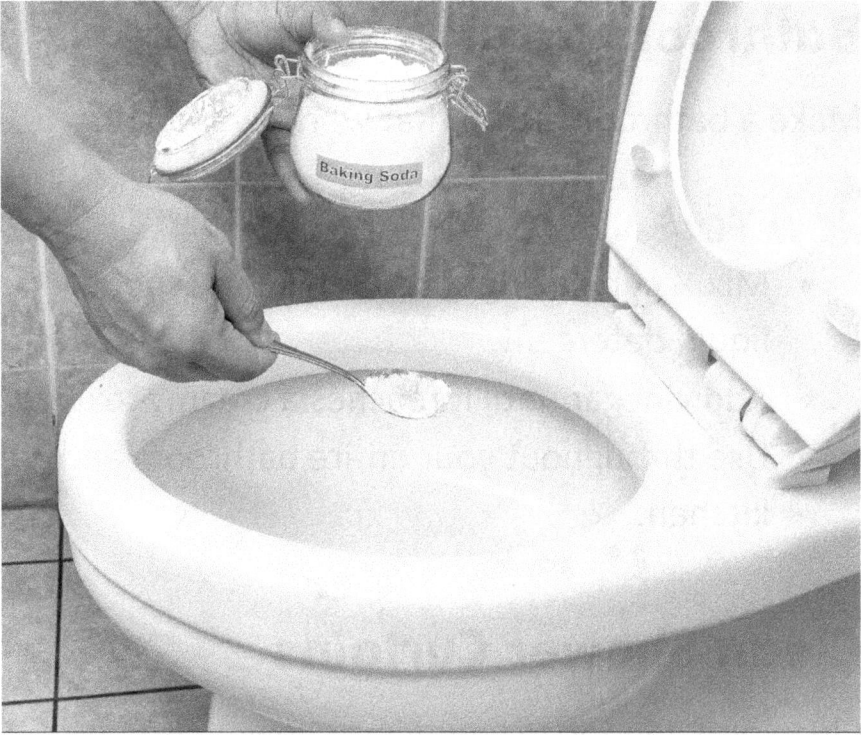

Bathroom

Bathroom Scrub

Make a bathroom scrub that works wonders.

How To:
- Mix ¼ cup baking soda with 1 tablespoon liquid detergent.
- Add vinegar until it reaches a creamy texture.
- Use throughout your entire bathroom and kitchen.

Clean Shower Curtains

Clean and deodorize your vinyl shower curtain.

How To:
- Sprinkling baking soda directly on a clean damp sponge or brush.
- Scrub the shower curtain.
- rinse clean.
- Hang it up to dry.

Clean Your Toothbrush

Many people overlook the need to clean their toothbrushes. However, many disgusting things thrive on this tiny wet bristle.

HOW TO:

- Add ¼ cup baking soda to ¼ cup water
- Let toothbrushes stand overnight.
- Rinse and use the next morning.

Mouth Appliance Cleaner

Soak oral appliances, like retainers, mouthpieces and dentures, in this amazing solution.

HOW TO:

- Dissolve 2 teaspoons of baking soda into a glass or small bowl of warm water.
- The baking soda loosens food particles and neutralizes odors to keep appliances fresh.
- You can also brush appliances clean using baking soda.

Septic Care

Regular use of baking soda in your drains can help keep your septic system flowing. It will help maintain a favorable pH in your septic tank.

HOW TO:

- Add 1 cup of baking soda into the toilet per week or add a toilet fizzy drop on a regular basis.

Toilet Fizzy Drops

Freshen things fast with toilet fizzy drops. They clean and eliminate smells immediately. Stash in a cute glass jar or container on the back of your toilet and simply drop in a fizzy when needed. It removes bad smells, clean your bowl, and is good for the septic. It's a miracle!

The next time things get smelly, after flushing, drop in a fizzy.

Ingredients:

- 1 cup baking soda
- 1/4 cup citric acid
- 1/2 teaspoon vinegar

- 1 tablespoon hydrogen peroxide
- 15 to 20 drops essential oil
- Sheet pan
- Parchment paper
- Measuring spoons
- Spray bottle (optional)

HOW TO:

- Add baking soda to a mixing bowl – break up any clumps.
- Add the citric acid.
- In a small glass bowl, mix together the vinegar and hydrogen peroxide.
- Now drop by drop, add the vinegar and hydrogen peroxide to the baking soda/citric acid mix. If you add the liquid all at once, you'll have a huge mess.
- Now add the essential oil and gently mix. Great options are wintergreen, lemongrass, or lavender.
- Use a ½ teaspoon to scoop and mold the mixture into small half rounds.
- tap the scoop onto a parchment-covered sheet pan.

- You can spritz the rounds with equal parts vinegar and water to create a crust, it helps hold them together.
- Let dry overnight.
- Place the dried fizzy drops in a sealable glass jar or sturdy container.
- Use as often as you would like.
- Makes around 30 small fizzy drops.

FYI: Its very decorative to place a label on the jar! And so that people don't think they are breath mints.

Unclog A Shower Head

HOW TO:
- Mix 1/3 cup of baking soda with 1 cup of white vinegar.
- Pour into a thick freezer plastic bag.
- Secure the bag over your dirty showerhead with a strong rubber band.
- Leave the bag on the showerhead for 24-48 hours.
- Remove the bag and wipe down with a warm cloth.

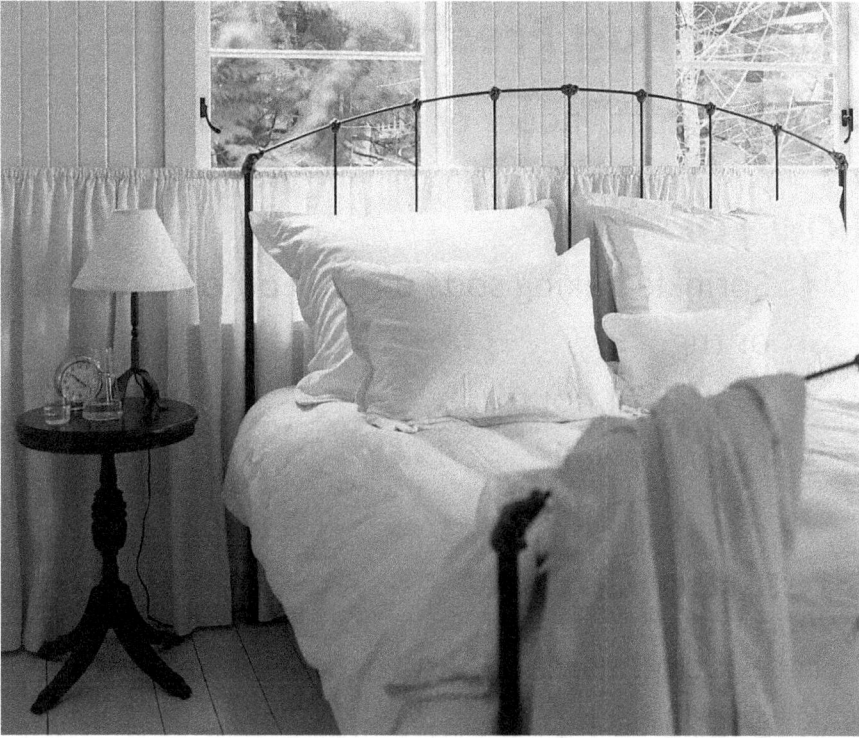

Bedroom

Carpet Rug Freshener

Freshen carpet, indoor or outdoor rugs.

HOW TO:
- Sprinkle baking soda directly onto the carpet or rug.
- Wait 2-24 hours.
- Vacuum well.

Freshen Closets

For fresh clothes, shoes and accessories use this baking soda trick.

HOW TO:
- Place a box on the shelf to keep the closet smelling fresh.

Freshen a Musty Mattress

Refresh your mattress with this trick.

HOW TO:
- Sprinkle all over your mattress.
- Leave on for up to 24 hours.

- Vacuum well.

Freshen Stuffed Animals

Keep favorite stuffed toys fresh with a dry shower of baking soda.

HOW TO:
- Sprinkle baking soda on each stuffed toy.
- Let sit for 1 hours.
- Vacuum, shake or brush it off.

Musty Book Makeover

Remove the musty funk from an old book.

HOW TO:
- Begin by dusting the pages lightly with baking soda
- Let it sit for 3-4 days.
- Shake, wipe or blow out with air.

Natural Jewelry Cleaner

Use a mix of water and baking soda to clean your jewelry.

HOW TO:

- Fill glass container with very warm water.
- Add 2 tablespoons of baking soda at a time until water becomes cloudy.
- Then drop in your jewelry.
- You can also use a soft bristle brush to remove grime.
- Rinse in cool water and pat dry.

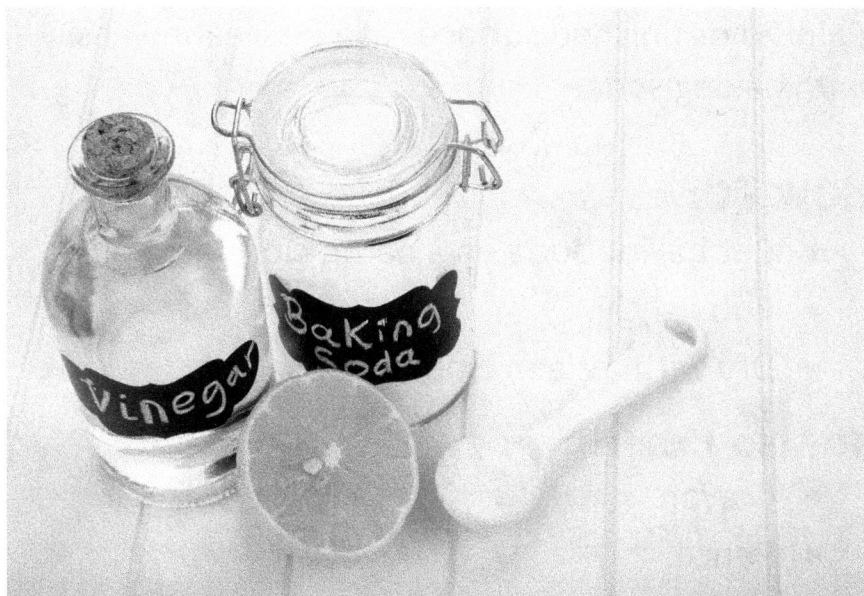

Furniture and Floor Cleaner

Painted or finished surfaces can be cleaned easily with baking soda.

How To:
- Put baking soda on a damp cloth or sponge.
- Rub lightly.
- Dry with a clean cloth.

It Also Erases:
- Crayon
- Pencil
- Ink
- Furniture scuffs from painted surfaces

Formica Cleaning Solution

Formica is another surface that can be loose its original shine with harsh cleaners. Use this easy to make solution to restore it to its former beauty.

How To:
- Add 3 tablespoons of baking soda to 1 quart of warm water.
- Gently wash using a soft sponge.
- Dry using a clean cloth.

Marble Solution

Properly cleaning marble countertops, furniture or floors can be challenging. This is a wonderful recipe that will bring back its luster.

HOW TO:
- Add 3 tablespoons of baking soda to 1 quart of warm water.
- Gently wash using a towel or soft sponge.
- Dry with a clean cloth.

Water Rings

Get rid of water rings on your tables with this mix.

HOW TO:
- Mix baking soda and toothpaste together well.
- Gently message the mix into the table in circular motions.
- When done wipe with a clean cloth.

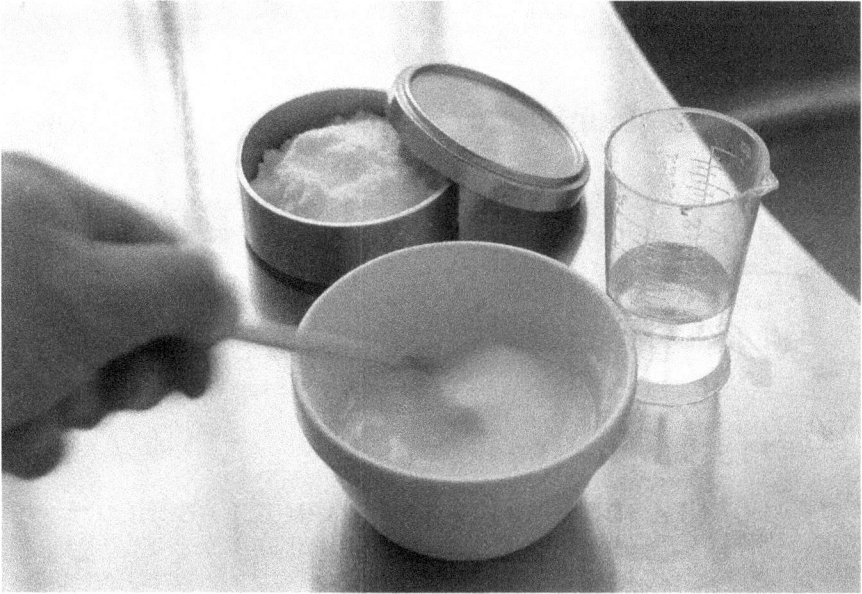

Home Improvement

Nail Hole Filler

Try this mix when you need to quickly fill nail holes in your walls.

How To:
- Mix baking soda and toothpaste together well.
- Press it into the nail hole.
- Let dry and touch up the paint if needed.

Spackle substitute

If you want to fill a small hole in plaster or drywall but would rather not purchase a whole tub of spackle for such a small job, try this odd tip:

How To:
- Mix baking soda and white toothpaste into a stiff paste.
- Apply it onto the area of concern.
- Let it sit for 1-3 days.
- Gently sand or apply touch up paint.

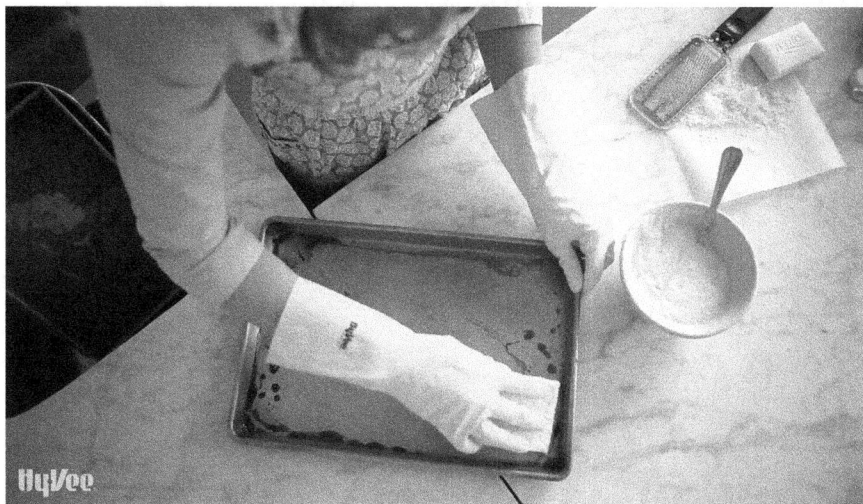

Kitchen

Ashtray Odor Stopper

This method eliminates the smell of heavily used ashtrays. The layer of soda traps the smoke from the ashes and discarded butts.

HOW TO:
- Fill the bottom of an ashtray with baking soda.
- Use as usual.

Baked on Grime

Everyone at one moment in time, makes a wonderful dish that destroys their nice pans. Don't soak for days and still never get it completely clean, use this wonderful and quick method.

HOW TO:
- Shake a generous amount of baking soda on entire surface.
- Add hot water and dish detergent.
- Let sit for 15 minutes and wash as usual.

Bring Back Lustre

To brighten a dull floor, try this gentle but effective solution.

HOW TO:

- Dissolve ½ cup baking soda in a bucket of warm water.
- Mop and rinse for a shiny floor.

Dishwasher Clean

HOW TO:

- Add 1 tablespoon of baking soda to the dishwasher.
- Run the dishwasher through a full cycle with NO dishes.
- When completed, use like normal.

Coffee-Pot Machine Clean

HOW TO:

- Fill your coffee pot with warm water.
- Add 1 tablespoon of baking soda to the water.

- Run the coffee-pot machine through a full cycle with NO coffee grounds.
- When completed, run another full cycle with water only.
- Then use like normal.

Shine Silver

This method allows you to shine tarnished silver on a dime.

How To:
- Combine three parts baking soda with one-part water.
- Rub onto silver with a clean cloth or sponge.
- Rinse thoroughly and dry.

Shine Brass, Chrome and Stainless Steel

You don't need a special polish for every surface in your home.

HOW TO:

- Use a damp cloth dipped in baking soda to clean and polish.
- Add a squirt of fresh lemon juice to brighten brass.

Deodorize the Cutting Board

If your cutting board is looking and smelling a little funky, this one is for you.

HOW TO:

- Sprinkle the cutting board with baking soda, scrub, rinse.
- Dry with a clean towel, let sit in an open-air location until completely dry.

Drain Deodorizer

Read caution before attempting this drain deodorizer. It is a very powerful cleaner!

Caution

- Use this method only if your pipes are <u>metal</u>.
- Never mix with other cleaning solutions.

- Don't use this if you have recently used a commercial drain product.

HOW TO:

- Pour ½ cup baking soda down the drain.
- Add ½ cup vinegar.
- After 15 minutes, pour hot/boiling water down the drain slowly.

Oven Cleaner Degreaser

Easy and non-toxic way to clean your oven.

HOW TO:

- Sprinkle baking soda in your oven and spray with water.
- Let it sit overnight.
- Mix a small bowl of warm water and a little dishwashing soap.
- Then scrub the oven and scoop out the clumped baking soda.

Remove Refrigerator Odor

This is the most common usage and the easiest way to keep your refrigerator smelling odorless.

HOW TO:

- Place an open box of baking soda in the door and leave.
- Bad smells are neutralized every day.

Trash Can Odor Control

Everyone has a trashcan that could use some odor control. This is a great way to tame the smell.

HOW TO:

- Sprinkle baking soda on the bottom of your trashcan.
- If you have discovered a leak in the bottom, sprinkle baking soda, dish washing soap, and hose it out in the yard.

Freshen Sponges

Sponges are often a forgotten source of germs. Clean often and well.

HOW TO:

- Mix 4 tablespoons of baking soda in 1 quart of warm water.

- Soak stale-smelling sponges for 4-6 hours.
- Rinse well with warm water and let sit in an open-air location until completely dry.

Clean the Microwave

This hack works on even the messiest microwave.

HOW TO:
- Put baking soda on a warm sponge or rage.
- Scrub inside and outside of the microwave.
- Rinse well with warm water.

Deodorize Recyclables

Use this trick to remove smells from reusable containers.

HOW TO:
- Mix baking soda and dishwashing soap together.
- Clean using warm water – do not use HOT water if working with plastics.
- Rinse well and dry.

Deodorize Garbage Disposals

It's important to deodorize your garbage disposals 1x per month or more.

HOW TO:
- Slowly pour ¼ cup of baking soda down the drain while running warm tap water.
- Turn on the disposal until all baking soda is washed away.
- Baking soda will neutralize odors for a fresh smelling sink.

Goo Remover

This Goo Remover works like magic, and it is completely food safe!

This Works On:
- Grease
- Stickers
- Remove labels
- Crayon
- Color Pencils
- And anything gooey

Ingredients

- ½ cup of olive oil or vegetable oil.
- 1/2 cup baking soda.
- Optional: add an essential oil if you would like. Many commercial cleaners use orange.

How To:

- Combine all ingredients in a jar.
- Shake well.
- Apply to surface.
- Let sit for 1 minute.
- Gently rub or scrub the goo.
- If extra gooey let it sit for up to 5 minutes before removing.
- Wash with hot soapy water.
- Dry with a clean cloth.

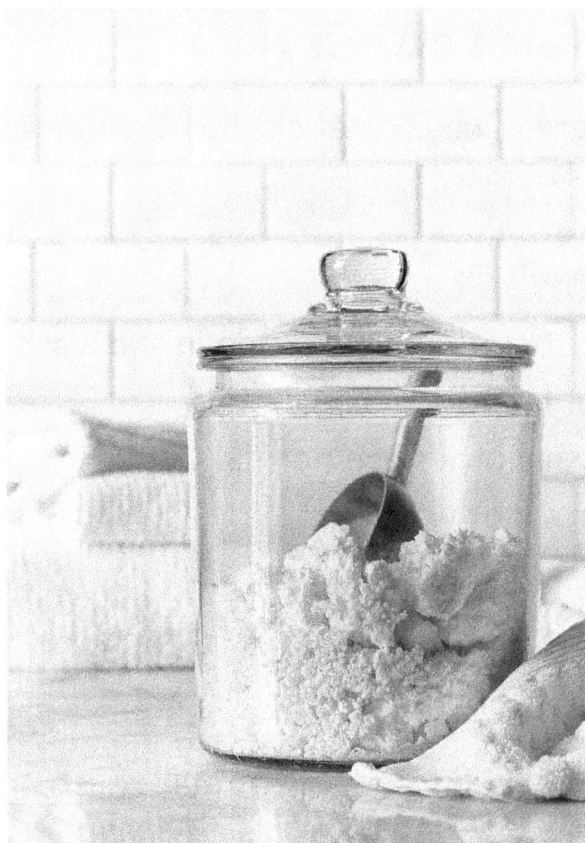

Laundry

Brighten Laundry

This is a great way to get clothes cleaner and brighter.

HOW TO:
- Add 1 cup of baking soda in the wash with your laundry detergent.
- Wash clothes like normal – for whites, use warm/hot water.

Canvas Handbag Cleaner

HOW TO:
- Apply baking soda on a small brush.
- Rub canvas handbag.
- If there are spots that are stained, use a small amount of water.

Clean Cloth Diapers

HOW TO:
- Dissolve 1/2 cup of baking soda in 2 quarts of water.
- Soak diapers thoroughly for up to 8 hours.
- Wash as usual.

Clean and Freshen Sports Gear

HOW TO:

- Mix 4 tablespoons baking soda in 1 quart warm water.
- Gently scrub or soak to deodorize smelly sports equipment.

Clothes Iron Cleaner

Remove all the residue from your iron, so you do not get stains on light colored clothing.

HOW TO:

- Mix a paste made from a little baking soda and vinegar.
- Gently rub onto the iron, making sure to avoid the holes.
- Wipe the mixture off with a warm damp cloth.

New Clothes Detox

Remove the harmful chemical finishes on new clothing.

How To:
- Add 1/2 cup of baking soda in the wash with your laundry detergent.
- Wash clothes like normal.

Rid Sneaker Smell

This trick will absorb the odor without making a mess or harming delicate materials like suede.

How To:
- Pour a few tablespoons into a paper coffee filter or sturdy tissue paper.
- Tie it up with a rubber band.
- Stick it into a stinky shoe.

Safely Clean Gold Irons

How To:
- Mix 3 parts baking soda to 1 part water.
- Use a cloth or soft bristle brush to clean.

- Rinse thoroughly.
- Pat dry with a clean cloth.

Stinky Hamper

Deodorize a funky-smelling hamper.

HOW TO:
- Sprinkle baking soda in the bottom of the hamper, or over the dirty clothes.

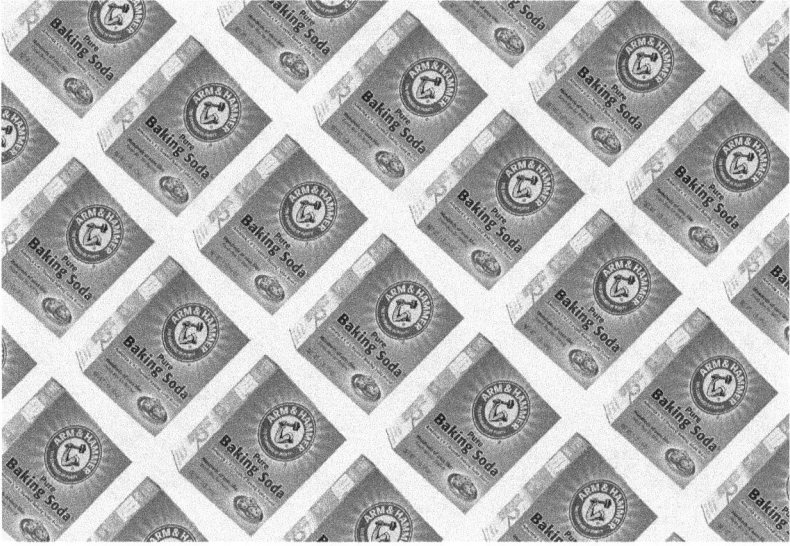

Oil & Grease

Absorbs Oil Grease, Juice, & Wine Stains

Works On:
- Carpet
- Rugs
- Upholstery
- Linens
- Drapes
- Blankets
- Concrete
- Hard floors
- Chair cushions and more...

HOW TO:
- Sprinkle a heavy amount directly on the liquid stain.
- Let the soda sit until the liquid has absorbed.
- Use a paper towel or dry cloth to remove the baking soda off the stained surface.
- Now you can use a warm wet cloth by itself, or a spot cleaner to remove left over residue.
- When completely dry, vacuum, wash or sweep the area well.

Grease Fire Extinguisher

If you ever have a grease fire, do not spray with water! Use baking soda instead.

HOW TO:

- You see a fire in the kitchen or garage.
- Get your baking soda box.
- Dump baking soda by the handfuls to extinguish flames.
- Call 911 as quick as possible.

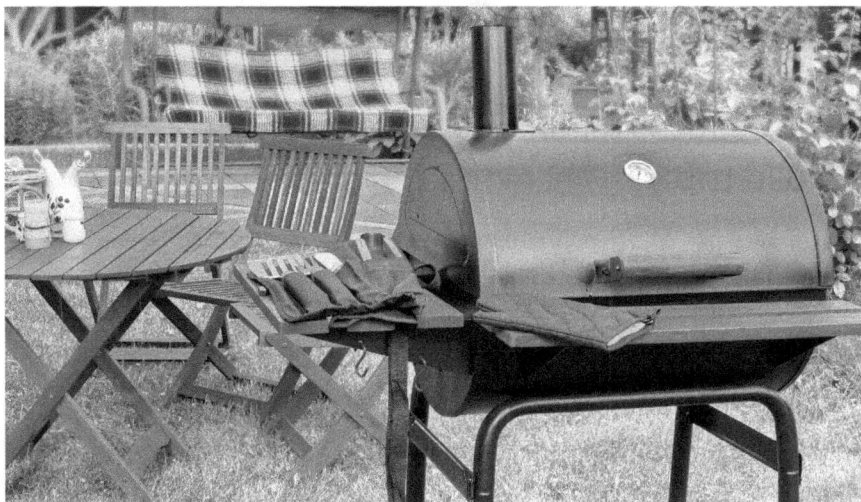

Outdoor

Camping Cure-all

Baking soda is a must-have for your next camping or road trip.

- ❖ It's a dish washer
- ❖ Pot scrubber
- ❖ Hand cleanser
- ❖ Deodorant
- ❖ Toothpaste
- ❖ Fire extinguisher

And many other uses...

Ice Cooler Odor Eliminator

Avoid that musty, moldy smell that camping equipment forms.

HOW TO:
- Sprinkle a bit of baking soda into your clean and dry cooler, thermos, and even tents before storing them away.

Grill Cleaning

Keep your grill clean all summer long.

HOW TO:

- Put some baking soda on a damp brush.
- Start scrubbing the grate.
- Then rinse well.

Patio Furniture

Before you store your patio furniture for the entire winter, try this solution.

HOW TO:

- Scatter baking soda under chair cushions.

Patio Furniture Sparkling Clean

Many times, cleaners are to abrasive to handle delicate outdoor furniture made from resin or plastic. They may easily scratch or dull the surface.

HOW TO:

- A wet sponge dipped in baking soda, will dissolve dirt without causing damage.

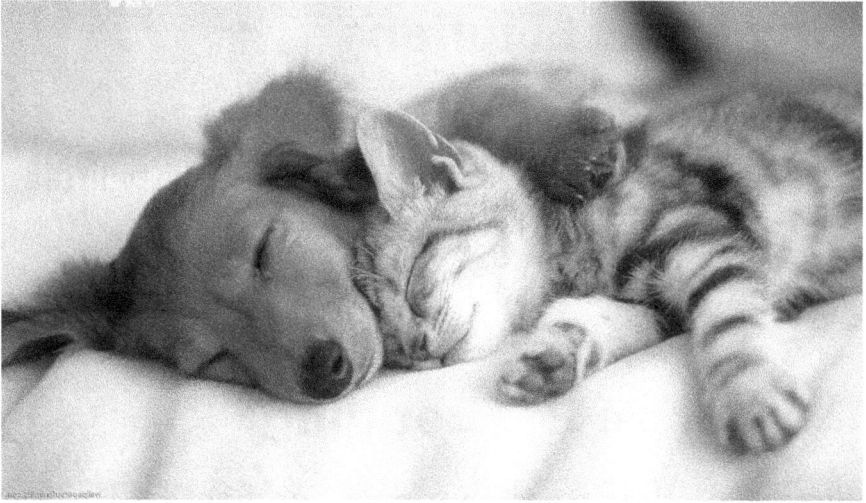

Pet Care

Kitty Litter Solutions

How To:

- Sprinkle baking soda in the empty kitty litter box.
- Add litter on top.

Deodorize Pet Bedding

Eliminate odors from your pets bedding.

How To:

- Sprinkle baking soda all over your pet's bedding.
- Let sit for 6 hours and shake out well.

Clean Brushes & Combs

Remove oil build-up and hair product grime.

How To:

- Start by soaking brushes in 1 teaspoon of baking soda and 2 cups of warm water for 1-4 hours.
- Rinse and allow to dry.

www.ingramcontent.com/pod-product-compliance
Lightning Source LLC
Chambersburg PA
CBHW060641280326
41933CB00012B/2103